TABLE OF CONTENTS

INTRODUCTION

If you are a parent or caregive, you are well aware that it can be challenging to care of small children. Moments of intense joy, closeness, and wonder may become perplexed and disturbed if the child appears mistaken or unhappy. You wonder what you can do to help your children stay happy and balanced.

Care for children is an effective strategy that helps children to build a deeper sense of self-awareness, emotional regulation, and focus. Any of the exercises are easy enough to do for anyone. For starters, during a short therapy session, children pay attention to various noises while listening carefully. Regular practice of attentive listening helps kids to relax before working on homework or other tasks.

DOES MEDITATION FOR CHILDREN REALLY HELP?

Most of the youths today spend their free time on internet electronic devices on different social media platforms, chatting and playing online games, and many more. Many experts agree that feelings of frustration, isolation, and disconnection will occur as such distractions overtake true interpersonal relationships and more imaginative and tactile pastimes. Indeed, "computer illness" has also been introduced to the classification of addicted mental wellbeing disorders by the International Health Organization.

Even children who are not married to their devices have difficulty balancing their school life, family life, social life, and personal time. They 're subject to the same feelings of stress and tiredness as adults. If not tested, stress build-up will culminate in a cascade of negative emotions.

Studies investigating the effect of mediation and mindfulness on the scholastic successes and children indicate that the activity contributes to greater attention, stronger performance, and enhanced memory. Carefulness helps kids stay grounded and savor the present moment. Helping them connect with their natural empathy and better understand their feelings has also been shown so they can manage them more effectively. This reinforces the sense of self-worth of children and gives them more room to express their innate creativity and compassion.

In reality, being conscious is one of the best gifts that we can give kids. It is a valuable resource and should continue to be incredibly helpful as they keep through. Many grown-up meditators wish they should have begun meditation sooner when their minds and bodies were more stable!

THREE GOOD MINDFULNESS TECHNIQUES FOR KIDS:

Mindful Breathing

Mindful breathing is just the same for children as it is for adults. Also, children are exposed to practice by an instructor or person who is already learning meditation. Children typically begin with a bit of controlled therapy to help them calm and concentrate, then spend a couple of minutes of breath awareness and finish up within a few minutes" – how do they express themselves? What, if anything, did they come across during this session? Are they any concerns about the procedure itself?

This attentive attitude – Tips meditation, silence awareness, and also check-in – was the same throughout whether the practices were directed on the breathing, seeking, or listening procedure. Note that during the last phase of practice, there are no right or wrong answers – this is not a test! Children, parents, and caregivers learn that they can recognize their experiences without feeling needing to react in one way or another.

Mindful Seeing

Mindful seeing strategies leverage the sense of seeing to help children develop a particular type of concentration. Usually, a tiny object is put in front of the children before the session starts. It may be a pebble, a stone, or some other visual anchor. This serves as the foundation of reflective reflection. Children must realize that the item chosen is an anchor for the mind to rest in so that it can relax and be present. It's not something that has to be debated or examined; it's not homework!

Mindful Listening

Mindful listening, like the previous two, is about having an attitude that isn't judgmental. Sound is the focal point of this situation. The progress here is again guided meditation, quiet listening, and check-in. Which one is that they've heard? Their heartbeats, birdsong, traffic, a lawnmower, a swallowing sound, a ringing phone, or a text message? Can such noises be described without the need to step on them? What does it feel?

How to introduce mindfulness to your children:

- ***Be good role models:*** Parents and guardians should set a precedent if they truly wish to encourage children to be conscious. When children see you meditating, they growing their interest and they want to pursue your lead and try it themselves.

- ***Make it simple and engaging:*** You don't want to find child care more difficult than that. Start utilizing strategies that would automatically catch your attention-it 's a perfect opportunity to listen carefully again. You may also use pictures and tales to speak about meditation.

- ***Encourage communication and feedback:*** Just like adults, when they meditate on children, they are likely to become more aware of their feelings. Invite your children to express what they have discovered; use this knowledge to connect freely, with reverence and approval.

- ***Make it fun:*** Kids want to play-who does n't? Render mindful exercise to look ahead from time to time, through adjusting emphasis. Take part in books and novels. Find a specific spot in your home that can be a nice relaxing corner for babies. Encourage the children to come along with their own drinks and prizes and help set them up. Create a "meditation cape" or "meditation blanket" that they can wear during mindfulness sessions – you could even make another one that you could use! Dream about what, if you had begun sooner, would have made mindfulness meditation special to you, which would have provided your children an incomparable gift about consciousness.

These are also perfect approaches to encourage children to meditate. There is a range of services available to help you and your child on your thoughtful trip.

WHY SHOULD WE TEACH KIDS MINDFULNESS?

The youth of today have a much more relaxed and isolated life than our parents or grandparents. Safety issues prevent parents from allowing their children to spend time outdoors under protection, as almost any generation has done before. The basic essence of American childhood has changed in a single century. The unstructured summer adolescence-days of cricket pick-up play, tree houses, and 'get home for dinner'-has all but disappeared."

Rather, children are overwhelmed with activities, ranging from kindergarten and music classes, sports leagues, language lessons, etc. Parents have to arrange to play dates to see other children outside the daycare, nursery or study, where children are allowed to interact with each other at someone's residence, indoor playground, or park for a certain amount of time with parents watching them.

Many children don't spend time outside, at least not the way children were required to do last year. Whitedog.org points out that riding has become 31 percent less common in the last 21 years (the National Sporting Goods Association and American Sports Data). Children are more likely enjoy to play video games instead of doing bikes riding (the Kaiser Family Foundation, also the CDC), and only 10 percent of American young children, who enjoyed playing video games instead of bikes riding.

Although not many people would argue about the need to keep our children safe and secure, especially in our day and age, this lack of freedom to spend time outdoors with friends, using their extra experience and goodwills, is creating children to lack a connection with their age mates and the global world as a whole.

Another problem is that since parents choose dates of play, children are surrounded by other children of similar race, ethnicity, and socioeconomic status who do not learn and appreciate diversity. This problem leads to a lack of sympathy, understanding, and acceptance and the ability of others to connect with people other than them.

What's the response to this issue? It's mindfulness in a word.

It began off as part of the Buddhist tradition, but over time it became a common practice known in the world. Practicing awareness involves being aware of the moment and accepting our mental processes (emotions, thoughts, reactions, feelings) and sensations of the body without classifying them as correct or incorrect or judging them. Mindfulness activities require reflecting on the here and now, rather than challenging our capabilities and worrying regarding previous failures or future uncertainty.

Mindfulness strategies allow one to concentrate on the moment and to become conscious of how and what we experience at the time. Mindfulness ensures that the past is finished and that the future has not yet taken place and allows us the "intention of staying in our memory."

By letting go of worry and focusing on here and now, we 're letting go of anger, frustration, irritation, annoyance and worry, and trying to achieve "equanimity — silence and balance of mind."

Why should we teach our kids mindfulness?

There are tremendous benefits for children to be mindful such as:

- Improved concentration
- Stress reduction
- Increased empathy
- Better mood
- Happier life
- Improved sleep
- More compassion
- Better self-awareness
- Decreased depression and anxiety
- An overall sense of well-being
- A deeper connection to nature
- A better understanding of energy
- Clearer thinking
- Loving-kindness
- Seeing beauty in others

GUIDES ON HOW TO PRACTICE MINDFULNESS FOR CHILDREN?

Start Simply - What's mindful in simple English? It's a tough subject for most people, and they understand it completely, so don't try and scare and intimidate your babies. Start by encouraging your little ones to practice meditation by reflecting on what they experience and are talking about. How quick are they able to breathe? What sort of emotions do they feel? Which thoughts are going through their minds?

Incorporate Daily Activities - Encourage the children to be involved at a moment when they're enjoying a family meal instead of scarfing their food. Ask them to smell and taste their food to describe the aromas and flavors. Through calming down and having the opportunity to eat meals, children can know how to calm down and concentrate more.

Use Toys - It recommends the use of toys that a child can put on his or her stomach while lying down. We 're going to focus on how the robot goes up and down as they breathe in and out. Give your little one the gift of true mindfulness, meditation, and yoga teddy bear, Meddy Teddy, instead of using some old toy. A flipping, rotating, and washable teddy bear allows parents to come to terms with the idea of mindfulness and how it will play a part in the child's existence. Plus, this little bear has a big message-he shares his positive thoughts on his own Instagram account.

FUN, EASY MINDFULNESS EXERCISES FOR KIDS

Consciousness has come up to attention in modern years as more of a social panacea. Current work shows us that interventions in mindfulness will reduce the effects of tension, anxiety, depression, and even physical pain. Mindfulness may also support individuals with intellectual difficulties, and cognitive conditions battle their condition's harmful consequences. What's more, due to its overall potential to promote healthy feelings and well-being, even people that aren't coping with physical, mental, or cognitive problems will benefit from attentiveness.

If you're a parent, you 're going to be glad to know that mindfulness works just as well for children as it does for adults. As children get older, they tend to cease living "at the moment" and become worried about their worries, hardships, and setbacks like adults. Exercises in mindfulness will help avoid this slow descent toward depressive thoughts and provide children with a greater cognitive and emotional understanding.

Children will, of course, be shown how to be careful with subtly changed strategies. The eight exercises below were adapted to reflect the average child's attention span:

1. Deep breathing

This is a great exercise to try and gradually settle for a nap when you want your child. Let your child be comfortable, then ask him to take a deep breath in and out. Ask him to describe how he feels when he enters his body, and when he leaves, have his breathing five times deep. Tell your child whose thoughts or emotions he is mindful of at a time when everything is going through. When his emotions or perceptions are pessimistic, he suggests believing that they are caught in bubbles. Finally, let him repeat a few deep breaths, instructing him to imagine "feeling bubbles" floating away as he does.

Sometimes very young children benefit from having a "breathing friend" to try the exercise. Place a favorite stuffed toy on your baby's stomach so that he can see and feel the effects of each deep breath more fully. Ask him to get her breathing mate and do deep breathing exercises together when your child is upset; it can help him calm, intense emotions.

2. Mindful posing

This exercise is a great way to help your child strengthen the relationship between body and mind. Ask your children to emulate their desired heroes (such as a Superman, Ninja, Spiderman, Monk, etc.) and then express to you how she/he feels about it while holding each pose. For added effect, let your child pretend that the super-powers increase their senses, then ask her what she can smell, hear, see, and taste.

3. The "feelings jar."

This exercise is both a fun craft and a useful tool to teach emotional consciousness. You 're going to need a brush, paint, and glitter glue to complete the build. (Other light waterproof decorations that are also "shakable" can be added.) Fill the container with water around three quarters, then apply a few soft glitter adhesives before closing the lid tightly. Let your child shake the jar and watch the glitter settle down in it.

When your child gets angry, worried, or upset, you can get her to take the jar off the shelf and shake her heart. Not only does the act of shaking the jar ease fear, but your child can also feel her feelings gradually settling down when she sees the glitter dropping. Tell your child that waiting for her feeling of relief will encourage her to think gradually and clearly, even though the water becomes eventually clear again as the glitter settles down on the bottom of the bottle.

4. The safari of the senses

The purpose of this activity is to help children completely engage in (and enjoy!) the present moment. Take your child out to imagine that she's in a safari. Ask her to be as silent and stealthy as possible so that she can watch any mammal, bird, and insect she sees without scaring them away. Encourage her to place her senses on high alert and notice little items she would usually overlook (like tiny insects in the grass).

5. Scent sensations
Collect a bunch of sweet-smelling items, such as fragrant candles, flowers, herbs, fruit, etc., and ask your child to breathe deeply into every fragrance. Take a moment to pause and ask your child what kind of emotions and memories this particular fragrance evokes. Sensory encounters such as these both anchor the child in a moment and allow him to become more mindful of his feelings and emotions.

6. Mindful strolling
Have your child calm down and concentrate on his breathing instead of running to classes, parks, and so on. Try to ask him what kind of things he sees, hears, and feels as he walks, like the smell of fresh air or the sound of the wind blowing through the leaves of the tree.

7. Slow snacks
Snacks offer another great time to slow down and fully experience the senses. Each time your child has sweets, remind him to detect food first when your child has a snack, then bite down and chew carefully, giving careful attention to the sound of chewing and the delicate variations of taste. You can always let your child stop at the end of the snack to concentrate on the rewarding sensation of fullness.

8. Meditation moments
While young children usually lack the patience required for any kind of guided meditation, older "crazy gadgets" children are likely to enjoy the free Smiling Minds meditation app (suitable for children seven and above). Alternatively, you can engage your child in a short meditation to keep her engaged. Making the moment more enjoyable by doing something that you still love having a pleasant one-on-one time with your boy.

9. Take a mindful walk
You can walk around the backyard or the neighborhood. Encourage younger children to be conscious by guiding them through their senses.
"What do you suggest this flower smell feels like when you walk? How do

you hear it? How do you feel it? How do you see it? Be truly present and pay attention to every moment," Pulikkiel suggests.

Older children and teenagers should use the audio device to direct them on a mindful trip.

10. Encourage Mindful Meals

Sit down and appreciate every aspect of a meal with your family. First of all, think about how thankful and happy you are for the food and the person who made it. Dream of serving dinner. What does that look like? Are they being served hot or cold? Whether you feed with your mouth or with silverware, be mindful of that. Think of the way it smells and the smell.

"Live your life at the moment and enjoy all the interaction," says Pulikkiel. "You don't need to do the whole meal. Some families have found that careful eating helps to reduce overeating because they are more aware when they're full."

11. Introduce The Idea of a Mindful "Body Scan"

You and your children can perform a careful body scan while standing up or sitting down. Some people in the mindfulness app use a guided audio clip.

Talk about every aspect of your body, start from above. The ultimate goal of body scanning is to help you relax and relieve stress by being in the present moment for a while.

"You desire and determination on every single part of your body. You can pull and relax every muscle when you breathe," says Pulikkiel. "Most importantly, the body is settling down."

Don't worry if when you're practicing awareness, your eyes are drifting to other subjects; that's natural!

"Just remember to come back to the moment and bring your attention back to your breath," says Pulikkiel. "Very frustrating for some youths; for the very first time, they are trying to make it right. Again, we 're reminding them that they're not courteous and friendly."

Body scanning may help young adults and twins deal with a bad self-image.

"Once again, we encourage them to be respectful to any aspect of their bodies and to be thankful for them," said Pulikkiel. "Showing Recognitions, thinking as it's without

overheating, it brings about a balanced outlook oneself."

PROMOTING MINDFULNESS IN KIDS

One of the most important recent development in the global treatment of sadness has been the side-effects of cognitive-behavioral principles.

Carrying out mindfulness is a way of meditation that emphasizes closing down depressive and negative thinking by paying close attention only to the present moment and following the things of your thoughts. Instead of striving to change the contents of your thoughts openly, mindfulness practitioners are developing the capacity to "bear witness" to them in a relaxed, non-judgmental way. Those who develop this discipline are often capable of breaking the stranglehold of the depressed state of mind.

Psychologists have tried to explain why an approach to mindfulness may be so successful. They believe that one of the main drivers of depressive thinking is obsessive "discrepancy analysis"—in other words, a concern about the seemingly insurmountable gap between where you are and where you would like to be. Their opinion is that the mindfulness approach has short-term effects these painful and counter-productive ways of comparison by not changing the present or focus beyond it, but by accommodating it for what it is, even if it is unpleasant to them.

The main reality is that our experiences change day by day, but a sad and depressed person usually ignores anything that might prove to be neutral uplifting. The practice of mindfulness leaves the patient exposed to reality in a way that is opposite to the routines of a troubled mind. It denies people from being caught up in the mind of negative thoughts by making everything simple and assisting people becoming more observers of their own thinking rather than been enslaved.

Research evidence shows that mindfulness practice may potentially help to reduce relapse in depressed adults, and core behaviors are also likely to support a psychologically healthy outlook.

Of course, we can encourage our children to develop some of the hallmarks of mindfulness. Learning to focus, to analyze, and to live in the moment is a skill that needs to be created. It begins with learning to keep the busy young minds babbling and bringing attention back to work at hand. The modern world leaves us in a constantly over-stimulated state: we are awash with information from the media and the Internet; our lives consist of ever-changing priorities and roles.

Encourage your child to focus, avoid obstacles, notice, and live in the present.

Since we have been used to coping with constant flux and so many competing demands, the ease and concentration of doing one thing at a time are becoming quite new to us. If the stimulus level falls below the cultural norm, often children feel ill at ease. Teach your child to be as confident with simplicity and quiet as it is with the pyrotechnics of the digital generation.

No one has been designed for multitasking all the time. How will your kid learn to take note of the tastes and textures of food while every meal is followed by the intrusion of the TV set? Go out with your children to enjoy natures and train him to observe: point out details and examine the intricate veins on the back of the leaf, also ridges on the shells or the glistening paths left by the snails. Sit together on the hillside; meditates together and see if you can focus on listening — Deep listening for a few minutes. Start encouraging them to do these things while your children are still young, and you will be building good mental hygiene for their later life.

Bring your kid out and let him/her learn the finer aspects of science. Help him/her learn how to be comfortable with simplicity and silence.

It's a shame that the craft of gathering items has been too overlooked. Either it is a stamp or bottle caps, putting over a prized collection help children to put their attention on things that are not supported by the fast-moving world of videos and computer games.

Recent health work shows us that the desire to function entirely at the moment and to establish a level of continuous care has a real preventive benefit on both of us.

The 17th-century French moralist Jean de la Bruyère claimed that "children have neither past nor future; they enjoy the present." However, although children may have an innate talent for "living in the current situation," we must have in mind that life is not stable its changes, making it more difficult to hold on to the precious ability. If you have made up your mind about protecting our child mental health ability, we must work
harder to get it done if we want our children to be able to succeed
 from the constant distractions of modern life.

WHAT ARE THE BENEFITS OF MINDFULNESS FOR CHILDREN?

There are many avenues that mindfulness will enhance everyone's mental well-being. But what are some of the advantages that are unique to children's everyday lives? First, awareness exercises are perfect for youngsters, as they:

- Easy to implement.

- Take time to implement.
- Are affordable.
- It can be performed anytime, at any moment. (In this book, mindfulness strategies are perfect for the home, school, and public spaces.)
- Funny! Incorporating pleasure increases the learning experience and lets children master the skills more easily.

Beyond this infrastructure, mindfulness provides many advantages for young people's bodies and minds. Let's take a deeper look at some of the physical and mental effects of youth.

Executive Functioning

The executive feature is a concept that involves many skills — work memory, perspective-taking, decision-making, emotional management, problem-solving, preparation, and impulse control. It sets the basis for all things relevant to education and culture. If children are under tension, good decisions make it more challenging for them to develop executive development skills. If the tension they encounter is persistent, the cognitive ability can be more severely affected, contributing to academic disabilities, performance loss, and behavioral disorders.

Work has shown that executive efficiency can be enhanced through mindfulness. This is because the regular practice of mindfulness consciously builds neural networks around the brain, creating associations and involuntary reactions. Consistent application in mindfulness improves the brain networks in synaptic superhighways, rendering cognitive activity more available to children through difficult periods. Just tell your classmate to take a toy from your brother, for example. Instead of screaming and getting it back (which may be caused by an old neuronal pathway), the child may immediately turn to the practice of mindfulness and take deep breaths before asking whether they could get the product they were using back.

BELOW ARE SOME RECOGNIZED BENEFITS THAT MINDFULNESS CAN PROVIDE FOR YOUR CHILDREN EXECUTIVE FUNCTIONING:

• Boosts of memory functioning (temporary storage and management of information on cognitive activities)

• Reduces impulsiveness
• Encourages management and capacity-building
• Gain the capacity to execute and supervise their own activities
• Promotes executive versatility (consideration of certain perspectives)
• Develops emotional wisdom (the capacity to sense and regulate one's own emotions)
• Strengthening competencies that lead to better decision-making

Mental Health
Simple mindfulness techniques like those in this book will offer resources to help children deal with any pain, frustration, and anxiety they face in their daily lives. Numerous study has also shown that teens with a variety of conditions – such as depression, anxiety, attention-deficit hyperactivity disorder, and eating disorders – gain from exercise responsiveness. Research has demonstrated that well-established activities in mindfulness can reduce the effects of these disorders and enable children to be relaxed, healthy, and satisfied.

LISTED BELOW ARE SOME RECOGNIZED BENEFITS THAT MINDFULNESS CAN PROVIDE FOR YOUR CHILDREN MENTAL HEALTH:
• Decreases depression and distress
• Increases concentration and attention
• Reduces negative self-confidence
• Improves happiness
• Ease depression symptoms
• Help to overcome somatic symptoms (psychological symptoms)
• Promotes conscious self-awareness
• Enhances social and emotional competences
• Enhances the ability to handle difficult emotions
• Reduces hyperactivity and attack
• Improves action management
• Decreases reactivity and encourages calm
• Enhances relaxation and peace of mind
• Relieves doubts and thoughts of impotence
• High and low energy balances
Always have one on one conversation with your child's health care providers, ask them about the most effective way you can manage your child's specific

conditions.

Well-Being

Mindfulness also has beneficial effects on the overall well-being of children. Research has shown that 10-minute daycare experience can have a relatively rapid impact on child protection. A rising child is special — children will learn different methods with growing practice and provide a complete toolbox within a few months that they can use in difficult times.

SOME RECOGNIZED BENEFITS THAT MINDFULNESS CAN PROVIDE FOR YOUR CHILD'S WELL-BEING:

- Improves self-esteem
- Supports attainment of personal goals
- Enhances empathy, optimism, persistence, and resiliency
- Promotes the development of social relationships
- Creates self-connection and self-awareness
- Expands connection with nature

Consistent interaction for your child can promote valuable social qualities, such as adaptability, compassion, and appreciation.

Learning

Mindfulness can also play a role in the growth of cognitive and academic skills. Improvements in learning performance and critical reasoning are related to the development of executive processing abilities. Mindfulness lets children concentrate on the tools they need to begin their mission, plan their job, identify the measures they need to accomplish their assignments and finish their goals. If children are attentive, they will offer attention, stick to tough situations, stop disturbances, and not get upset.

HOW MINDFULNESS CAN BENEFIT YOUR CHILDREN LEARNING. MINDFULNESS:

- Expands metacognition (essentially thinking).
- Improves academic success.
- Facilitate anxiety testing.
- Boosts imagination.
- Implements with a more efficient application of information.

• Enriches knowledge and insight in thought.
• Strengthens attitude that helps fine motor functions, including blogging.
• Promotes better working standards and teamwork.
• Raises the enrollment rate at college.

A lot of things affect academic success, but the practice of mindfulness is likely to provide children with strategies that can be adapted across their life and the way they perform education.

Physical Health

Work has demonstrated that awareness can help children keep healthy and make better decisions regarding their health issues. Consciousness about eating and nutritional choices can, in particular, affect the physical health of the child, now and later as an adult.

REGARDING YOUR CHILD'S HEALTH, STUDIES SHOW THAT MINDFULNESS:

• Reduces blood pressure
• Improves and eliminates digestion
• Bolsters the immune response
• Helps do easier
• Aiding serious disease
• Heightens body awareness and engine planning
• Improves sense integration
• Reduces stress hormones, for example, cortisol

Considering The Social-Emotional Benefits Of Mindfulness

Why are we teaching thoughtfulness in our schools? The Scholarly, Social, and Emotional Learning Collaborative (CASEL) works on two main socio-emotional competencies: self-regulation and self-awareness. Skills in these areas not only teach students how to understand their thoughts, attitudes, and behaviors but also how to react positively to them.

Practicing mindfulness can alter the brain structure in a way that can improve a student's response to stress, according to brain imaging research. It densifies the prefrontal cortex, which is responsible for vision and thinking and improves blood supply throughout the brain. And calming therapy not only decreases the intensity of tension but may also serve to ease anxiety or depression.

If discrimination is a big issue at your office, it could be a great chance for your classroom to demonstrate thoughtfulness. Research shows that the level of violence in schools offering mindfulness exercises is considerably lower. As students begin to understand their feelings and positively respond to them, they are less likely to strike at their peers.

The last reason to check your intelligence in the classroom? Children with learning disabilities, specifically attention deficit hyperactivity disorder (ADHD), may be particularly helpful. The research found out that children with disabilities who have been educated in mindfulness had benefited better and had fewer emotional distress than when the program began. Carefulness will also enable children with special needs to improve social-emotional skills that can help them communicate with peers.

Finally, for every child in your community, mindfulness has something to give. It can relieve student stress, reduce the rate of abuse, and encourage children with learning disabilities or special needs to develop better SEL skills. If you haven't done the class learning exercises yet, now may be the opportunity to see how much your students can benefit from.

TECHNIQUES TO USE DURING CHILDREN MINDFULNESS TRAINING

1. Techniques to Use with Infants

You might not think that tiny babies would know what's going on ... Much less do you grasp a major idea, like being conscious?

Although babies may not be able to express their emotions with anything but tears, children from 6 to 8 weeks of age can understand the voices and scents of their parents. In this era, mindfulness can be about the stimulation of the emerging senses.

But, at this point, it will more be about getting you more conscious of yourself as a parent so that you can help your child understand it when they grow up.

Practicing a daily infant massage with your baby may be one way to start a practice of mindfulness. To continue with, wait about 45 minutes after feeding so that your kid doesn't spit milk. Change the child's indications — notice if they're quiet, warning, or agitated.

Massage your kid under gentle pressure. You should start on their stomach and then work the head, neck, shoulders, and other parts of the body in each position for about a minute — a minimum of 5-10 minutes. Slowly and gently, pay attention to how your little one reacts to your look and your touch.

Possible effects of child massage investigated can involve improved attachment between the baby and the caregiver, stronger sleep/relaxation, healthy hormone boosts to regulate pain, and decreased crying.

THE OLD CHILDHOOD DEVELOPMENT NONPROFIT ORGANIZATION ZERO TO THREE-POINT OUT FEW OTHER TECHNIQUES FOR BETTER CONNECTING WITH YOUR BABY IN A MINDFUL WAY:

• **Pay full attention to your baby**: It's not about neglecting your own desires. But as you communicate, seek to look into the environment, your baby's attitude, their physical health, and whatever other hints they send you to how they behave.

• **Put yourself in shoes for your baby:** Respond to their cries and indignation at love and humility — how would you like to be treated if you shouted!

• **Accept parental sentiments:** Sleepless nights can be rough, so getting fully spent is perfect. Don't find yourself less than positive for being incredibly sleepy. Sometimes, remember to tell yourself that your kid doesn't sit awake to punish you through the night.

2. Techniques to Use with Toddlers and Preschoolers

Are you going to meditate for a 3-year-old? Maybe not. Children in this age range are all about exploring limits and achieving freedom. This involves a lot of tantrums and difficult times for parents and tots alike. You have learned more about the "Terrible Two."

Before behaving destructively, cognitive techniques for the tots revolve through the senses to encourage children to understand what they experience within.

Model mindfulness

One of the best places to set out on this journey is to practice your mindfulness. Children learn from their environment, particularly their carers. If you are capable of modeling sensitivity and non-judgment, it can have a huge effect on your infant.

Activity:

Focus on some of the activities you do every day, such as bathing your child.

Experience the warmth of water between your hands and your smooth shower. Drink on the child's scents of the bath bombs and the sounds swirling about. Pay attention to the motions you create with your towel when you dry your boy.

Instead, you can only take five minutes a day and close your eyes and concentrate on breathing. Whenever your mind wanders, do your hardest to focus back on your inhalations and exhalations.

Provide language

People of this generation don't learn how to communicate their feelings orally. Give them the words to express what they feel in a way that you will understand. This makes young children pay heed and respect their inner feelings.

With time, the hope is that your child will express his or her emotions, or at least have the capacity to understand and deal with them.

Activity:

If your 3-year-old throws a block across the room, avoid being immediately labeled as bad. Or — more importantly — not to portray the child as evil.

But, you might suggest something like, "I see you've got a lot of strength right now. We can't throw stuff into your house ... but let's find another way out of your wiggles.

This approach helps to prove to children that their actions are not inherently bad. It can help them recognize when they feel extra active in the future and provide options for better energy recovery.

Focus on the senses

Although young children do not grasp all brain behaviors when they contribute to cognition, they do benefit from the cycle of experiential learning. So, instead of presenting mindfulness as some abstract concept, try to focus on the senses.

The tot doesn't know that listening to ocean waves crashing along the shoreline helps to quiet them down. However, they do connect the connections to practice.

Activity: Take a nature walk out with your child. Let your little one know as the leaves shift through the wind. Direct your attention to the warm sun as it bathes your face. Listen to the birds chirping sound.

Focusing on the world lets the child interact with their surroundings. It's bringing them here and now to their attention.

Facilitate Body/Mind Awareness

If you ask a young child how they feel, they can immediately answer "healthy," or else they don't know. You will also allow them to check in with their bodies and minds by having them do a "body scan" where they pay attention to each area and then turn to the next one, noticing feelings or thoughts along the way.

Activity:

Encourage your little ones to talk about how they look, from head to toe. It may be a nice way to start a day or even something you do when you know your child wants to concentrate on himself.

If you encounter a stressful point in the future-turn your child back to body scanning; will they feel tight in their tummy, or are they nervous in their shoulders? Explore these places and also figure on strategies to calm using certain methods, such as deep breathing.

3. Techniques To Use With Elementary School-Age Kids

Grade school kids struggle with multiple challenges at home and at school that test their feelings, focus, and willingness to cope with themselves. Now that children have more words, techniques may be better employed to promote their practice of mindfulness.

Experts at Concordia University explain that when children of this age feel overwhelmed, they can step back now and ask themselves questions like, "Am I confused? Hungry? Crazy? Do I need to breathe?

Guided imagery

When they get older, school children can have issues with conventional meditation. Using guided photo exercises allows them to bring their mind to their feelings and a safe way to relax.

Seek experimenting with something quick and improving over time as your child transitions to the schedule if your child has trouble over lengthy workouts.

Activity: YouTube has a wealth of video footage for both children and adults. Johns Hopkins, for example, offers a 15-minute sea-themed exercise in which children can either close their eyes to participate or keep them open and soak up in the fishy scenes. The narrator asks the children to look at how they look, and to visualize the swim with the rays. There are also moments of silence that allow for quiet breathing and self-reflection.

Yoga

Connecting breath and body movement will help bring the consciousness of your child to the present moment. Yoga can be a relaxing way to help wiggle out when adding different forms of meditation, such as deep breathing, into the mix.

Activity: Check out your area and see if anyone offers organized yoga for children. But you can also do this at school, free of charge.

Cosmic Kids Yoga has a large collection of yoga activities for kids of all ages three and above. They also offer "Zen Den" videos that encourage positive thinking and focus, such as Superpower Listening.

If you want to try yoga, make sure the distraction-free practice (think of clutter-free and dim lighting) provides a healthy and relaxing spot.

Mindful Eating

Eating is the experience of a sensory nature. Children see the food right in front of them. They perceive its aroma and can consume their flavor. They can also detect the food's texture in their tongues.

Careful eating can help children of school age create stamina for quietness and focus. And it might just as well be a fun way to use snack time thoughtfully. (Adults should even practice healthy eating!)

Activity: Gather any items, such as a timer, a slice of sugar, or a pinch of raisins. Close your child's eyes, and put the food inside your mouth. Tell him not to chew it, to concentrate on food.

If you are using something melty, like a slice of chocolate, make them concentrate for a few minutes on melting it in their mouth. If you feel their thoughts are changing, try to restore them to the sweet melting or texture of the raisin, all bumpy on their tongue.

Stillness Practice

Another way of encouraging stillness is to play a little bit with the idea. That technique can be fun at home as well as in the classroom. At first, children can have trouble staying calmly over a long time, so suggest setting a timer to start with just 2 minutes and attempting to build your way up to 30 minutes overtime.

You might even find it amusing to track your child's progress on a chart so they can feel a sense of accomplishment as they progress.

Activity: Sit your child in a comfortable position, maybe crossed legs or the lotus yoga position. Dim the lights, and play soothing music. Start the timer and encourage your child to turn a blind eye and focus on breathing or music. Try to remind them to stay calm, breathe, and stay still if they fidget or are having trouble. When it's almost time to stop, encourage them to begin slowly wiggling their fingers and toes to help bring awareness back into their bodies. And then stretch out and discuss how that went.

4. Techniques To Use With Tweens And Teens
Many of these same techniques are still useful as children get older (and even young adults). Karen Bluth, an expert and attentiveness instructor, says that at this age, children can be particularly suspicious and even resistant to attempting strategies of attentiveness.

Tips:

- **Space matters:** Bluth taught at-risk teenagers various techniques and said their overall experience was influenced by the room where teenagers were practicing. Relax in a room that produces no negative emotions. In this case, the move from a classroom to a gym was necessary. This may involve moving away from your siblings or mobile devices into a quiet space within your home.

- **Play it cool:** Teens may not want to be told to try the techniques of being aware of it. Instead, it's good that the idea is presented to them, and they can choose whether they want to participate or not. The idea may be pushing backfire. Suggest it gently.

- **Model:** It's important to practice what you're preaching ... even with the set of tween/teen. If your child is especially resistant to the idea, try not to judge at all. Bluth quoted "know when they are ready, they will be involved."

- **Try a variety of techniques:** If simple meditation doesn't fit your child, there are other choices to provide, such as yoga, body scanning, relaxation techniques, or directed imaging. The actual approach doesn't care so much as the ability to reach your child.

Note:

The research so far on teaching children's knowledge has mainly been achieved by structured activities, typically in a therapy (and probably school) environment. But teaching these principles to your children can very well be beneficial to you as a parent.

In reality, integrating mindfulness techniques into daily life can have powerful effects on your child — and your family culture as a whole. If there is one technique that does not speak to your little one, try another. Every person is different, so your 4-year-old or tween may not find what works for you as compelling.

The most important part of the process is to keep the experience consistent and positive. With time, the ability of your child to connect with itself and its surroundings should grow and flourish.

TOP 100+ MINDFULNESS RESOURCES FOR CHILDREN AND TEENS

In basic terms, mindfulness is the process of being conscious of something and concentrating your thoughts on the current moment. When you practice mindfulness, you are calmly conscious of your thoughts and feelings.

Mindfulness, as a practice, is not for adults. Children and adolescents can benefit from this, as well.

Here's a list of useful apps, books, and videos to share with your kids and teens to help bring the concept and practice of mindfulness to your home and classroom.

A. Apps

1. Insight Timer

Free daily meditation practice with over 30.000 titles, the world's largest collection of free guided meditations. Child topics include meditation and sleep.

2. Calm

Calm is an app for meditation, sleep, and relaxation that helps listeners experience the amazing benefits of being mindful. The app contains sleep stories as well as guided meditations.

3. Headspace
The mission of Headspace is to improve global health and happiness. Users will learn the meditation and carefulness essential.

4. Waking Up
Check out these children's guided meditations. The recordings are intended for children aged between six and ten. Teens are allowed to use the Waking Up software here.

5. Smiling Mind App
Smiling Mind is an app developed by psychologists and educators for free mindfulness meditation. The programs are designed to help people tackle the pressure, stress, and challenges of everyday life.

6. Breathe, Think, Do with Sesame
This software demonstrates skills such as problem-solving, self-control, preparation, and execution with assignments. The research-based device, this bilingual (English and Spanish), lets your child learn Sesame's "Breathe, Reflect, Perform" problem-solving method. Children love acquiring dumb mental language, a method of controlled breathing, tailored motivation, and more!

B. Books for Children
7. Alphabreaths: The ABCs of Mindful Breathing
Alphabreaths: The Mindful Breathing ABCs by Christopher Willard and Daniel Rechtschaffen

In Alphabreaths, children practice their ABCs and the fundamentals of mindfulness by imaginative relaxation activities. Furthermore, playful, and delightful illustrations, Alphabreaths is the exact introduction to mindfulness and awareness of the breath.

8. Breathe Like a Bear
Breathe Like a Bear by Kira Willey
This direct illustrated collection of exercises on mindfulness is direct to teach

children techniques to maintain their bodies, breath, and emotions too.

9. A Handful of Quiet:
Joy in Four Pebbles
A Handful of Quiet: Joy in Four Pebbles by Thich Nhat Hanh
Pebble mediation is a friendly and interactive practice that parents and educators should do to expose them to mediation. It is structured to engage children in a hands-on and imaginative manner that enhances their relation to nature.

10. Stand Rigid Like a Mountain
Stand Rigid Like a Mountain by Suzy Reading
Children are natural masters of curiosity and attentiveness; therefore, learning is not a one-way street. The book helps parents to search for ways to benefit from their kids too.

11. Sitting Like a Frog
Sitting Like a Frog by Eline Snel
The book includes eleven activities that rely exclusively on these situations, complete with brief explanations and anecdotes.

12. I Am Yoga
I Am Yoga by Susan Verde
I'm Yoga encourages children to express the world of yoga exercise and make space in their hearts for the world beyond. A child-friendly guide to 17 yoga poses is included.

13. I Breathe
I Breathe by Susie Brooks
Using their imaginations, children are invited to seek depicted child-friendly yoga poses and relaxation exercises intended to help them regulate their emotions.

14. Matt's Swirly World
Matt's Swirly World by Madeleine Matthews
An amusing story starring a mother and her young music, this book is a wonderful example of how all feelings are valued and how positive behavior can be experienced by children and reinforced by carers.

15. Slumberkins
Slumberkins Series by Slumberkins
Our stories use research-based techniques to teach children important social-emotional skills. Although proactive and supportive narratives, each collection is intentionally crafted to build a resilient, caring, and confident child.

16. Silence
Silence by Lemniscates
This book helps children to sit, listen, and comment on their perceptions and the environment around them.
Using the characteristics of mindfulness and quiet reflection, readers are asked to pay heed to what is actually forgotten in our busy environments.

18. What Signify to be Present
What Does it Mean to be Present? by Rana DiOrio
Follow a group of friends at school, at home, and on the beach as they experience what it means to be present.

19. Take the Time
Take the Time by Maud Roegiers
This thoughtful and peaceful book encourages children to slow down and become conscious of their day-to-day actions and thoughts. With reassuring imagery and gentle rhythms, children may be directed to quiet self-awareness and mindfulness.

20. I am Peace
I'm Peace by Susan Verde and Peter H. Reynolds
This thoughtful and peaceful book encourages children to slow down and become conscious of their daily actions and thoughts. With gentle rhythms and calming pictures, children may be directed to calm self-awareness and mindfulness.

21. Puppy Mind
Puppy Mind by Andrew Jordan Nance
In this picture book, a small boy learns that his imagination is like a dog, constantly running away, in the past or in the future. By learning to relax, the boy is a happier and more loving owner of his puppy mind, holding him in the now, if just for a moment.

22. I Can Handle It

I Can Handle It! by Laurie Wright

Parents and teachers are astounded when children begin to say, 'I can do it' almost immediately after reading this novel! In stressful circumstances that normally trigger meltdowns, children tend to understand that they can fix challenges and potentially 'do' the crisis themselves.

23. I Matter

I Matter (Mindful Mantras) by Laurie Wright

Elise is a smart little girl who stops considering her own feelings only and realizes that she is most valuable and that she is MATTERS. Kids belong to their families and friends, and to the environment around them, so they deserve to learn.

24. Charlotte and the Quiet Place

The Charlotte and the Quiet Place by Deborah Sosin

Often kids need a break from our busy, over-stimulating culture. This book illustrates how an infant discovers and performs controlled breathing on its own and recognizes the value of quiet. All children should be interested in the ongoing journey and the lesson of self-discovery and encouragement.

25. My Magic Breath

My Magic Breath: Finding Calm by Nick Ortner's Mindful Breathing

In an environment that is still so noisy, with so many issues going on, My Divine Breath can help lead children through a serene place of concentration, self-awareness, and harmony.

26. Breathing Makes it Better

The Book of Sad Days, Mad Days, Glad Days, and all the Feelings In-Between by Christopher Willard

With rhythmic writing and attractive illustrations, this book guides children to breathe through their emotions and to find peace with recurring cues to stop and breathe. Easily directed interventions show children how to implement the principles of mindfulness as they need them most.

27. Bee Still

Bee Still by Frank Silio

Research has shown that meditation can help improve concentration and focus, soothe anxiety, and reduce impulsivity. Bee Still is a loving child introduced to meditation.

28. Mind Bubbles
Mind Bubbles by Heather Krantz
The book is a straightforward, descriptive, and positive definition of mindfulness that children aged 4-8 can appreciate and continue to explore for themselves. It can be read by or to young children and includes a guided, thoughtful breathing script for teachers and parents to read so that everyone can practice their new skills.

29. Wild Mindfulness
Wild Mindfulness by Laura Larson
This picture book is intended to educate, encourage and enable children (and adults!) to observe reflective moments by directed visualization and relaxation exercises as they follow along with a young girl and her adventures camping and exploring in the forest.

30. A World of Pausabilities
A World of Pausabilities by Frank Silio
Everyone can be mindful, including (especially!) kids. This tale is a gentle reminder to stop, take a break, and notice the most important things as we go through our busy days. Even the easiest moments are the most important — if we don't let them slip by!

31. Here and Now
Here and Now by Julia Denos
The benefit of identity and connection, inspire curiosity, and engage quick discussions about things of life.

32. Mindfulness for Kids
Mindfulness Exercises for Compassion, Concentration, and Relaxation
The boxed card set includes 50 imaginative mindfulness simulations, visualizations, and activities divided into five categories to help children feel centered, achieve peace of mind, improve focus, practice loving-kindness, and calming.

33. Relax Kids
A collection of books, audiobooks, and other products designed to help

children become resilient and provide them with tools and techniques to manage their emotional and mental health.

C. Books for Teens
34. Practicing Mindfulness
Practicing Mindfulness by Matthew Sokolov
With over 75 critical meditations — which take about 5-20 minutes from start to finish — Practical Mindfulness is an approachable way to incorporate mindfulness throughout daily life.

35. Mindfulness for Youth in 10 Minutes a Day
Mindfulness for Youth in 10 Minutes a Day by Jennie Marie Battistin
This book features simple and effective exercises — which fit perfectly into the daily routine — making it easy to keep in the here and now, to tackle challenges one at a time, and to make the most of every minute.

36. The Mindfulness Journal for Teens
The Youth Mindfulness Journal by Jennie Marie Battistin
This platform includes valuable techniques — simple relaxation strategies, quick reflection, and journal reminders to help alleviate tension and live in a moment.

37. 5-Minute Mindfulness Meditations for Teens
5-Minute Mindfulness Meditations by Nicole Libin for Teenagers
This book provides simple, fast activities that encourage you to utilize the power of mindfulness meditation — to pay careful attention to your body and your thoughts. These exercises, designed for real-world situations, teach readers to think and respond rather than react.

38. The Mindful Teen
The Mindful Teen by Dzung X. Vo
It is a groundbreaking curriculum focused on attention-related stress management (MBSR) and mindfulness-based cognitive therapy (MBCT) to help teenagers cope with tension. Simple, practical, and easy-to-remember tips in this book can be used every day to help manage any difficult situation more effectively.

39. Mindful Games Activity Cards

Mindful Game Activities Cards by Susan Kaiser Greenland
A group of 55 children's mindfulness games that a playful approach to build attention and focus, and emotional regulation.

40. Be Mindful Card Deek for Youths
Be Mindful Card for youths by Gina M. Biegel
These cards offer 50 ways of presenting themselves as life as it takes place. Teens can use these strategies of daily mindfulness when they feel anxious, moody, angry, or simply need to relax.

41. Mindfulness for Teen Worry
Mindfulness for Teen Worry by Jeffrey Bernstein
This book shows teenagers how living in the moment will dissolve worries and help them to remain grounded in the here and now. They will learn powerful and user-friendly attentiveness skills to manage the face of teenagers' four most common worry struggles.

D. Videos
42. Cosmic Kids Yoga
Cosmic Kids Yoga
Yoga, child care, and relaxation. Interactive experiences are creating strength, health, and confidence-and early yoga and mindfulness for youngsters!

43. 20 Minute Yoga for Teen with Nicole Cardoza
20 Minute Yoga for Teen with Nicole Cardoza
Join Nicole Cardoza, in practice, specifically designed to teach young people how to pay attention to their bodies, also to the world around them.

44. The Power of Concentrating Attention Nicole Cardoza TedX
The Power of concentrating Attention by TedX
Watch the Yoga Foster founder discuss her mission in schools to promote accessible, sustainable yoga programs. It aims to empower teachers to create healthier, happier classrooms.

45. 3 Minutes Body Scan Meditation
3 Minutes Body Scan Meditation by Fablefy
Children, parents, and educators love this meditation on body scanning. Shamash Alidina describes the body scan in Mindfulness for Kids as a way of getting in touch with the body, letting go of feelings of needing to get things done, and releasing pent-up emotions.

46. Cosmic Kids Zen Den
Zen Den Playlist-The Cosmic Kids Mindfulness Series
Learn how to make good choices using the traffic light technique. Stop-Breathe-Pick! Children have plenty of decisions to create every day-how do they and others make life easier for themselves?

47. Five Mindfulness Exercises for Kids
Five Mindfulness Exercises for Kids by Cosmic Kids
Five Easy and practical techniques of attentiveness for children over five years of age can be used to self-regulate, calm down, adjust their hearing, and sharpen their concentration.

48. Mindfulness for Teens
Mindfulness For Youth Voices by Kelty Mental Health
These video features youth and young adults discussing their conscientious experiences and how awareness have benefited various aspects of their lives

49. Everyday Mindfulness About Kids Health
Everyday Mindfulness About Kids Health
This video describes what situational consciousness is and how understanding what's going on around you and inside of you will actually make life more fun and less stressful.

50. Mindfulness for Teens and Adults Fablefy
Mindfulness for Teens and Adults by Fablefy
The main objective of mountain meditation is to get centered and reach our inner strength and stability when confronted with both internal, external stressful and challenging circumstances around them.

E. Other Mindfulness Activities For Kids
51. Heartbeat Exercise
When the students track their pulse, and during workout movement, they can grow to be conscious of how their body feels.

52. Pinwheel Breathing
This exercise helps students use a pinwheel to show them how to practice deep breaths.

53. Muscle Relaxation
How often do we really bear in mind the muscles in our bodies? With this

exercise, children may continue to learn, thinking of whether their muscles are tensed or relaxed.

54. Mindful Coloring
You should use printable sheets for a thoughtful coloring exercise that can be conveniently located online.

55. Five Senses Exercise
Were you aware that all five of your senses can be used while you are mindful? This can show you how!

56. The Present Moment Worksheet
This worksheet on free mindfulness teaches young students everything about what it means to be present.

57. Yoga for Kids
Check out this footage of a social mindfulness activity that will support elementary kids by age-appropriate and creative games to learn yoga.

58. Contentment Thermometer
Being mindful of our emotions is a key component of being mindful. This 'thermometer of contentment' can help students to define and track their feelings

59. Making Mindful Observations
Fill your science lessons with a little social-emotional learning by teaching students to make careful observations.

60. Teaching STOP Mindfulness
Teach children the key components of mindfulness by way of the acronym Rest: Rest, Relax, Listen, and Go.

61. Breathing Boards
Let the students follow the thread, taking steady, calculated breaths with their finger.

62. Gift of You
This festive activity is an excellent way to teach attention throughout the holidays.

63. Mindful Glitter Jar

This cute art will provide students with a tangible representation of how their emotions relax after practicing mindfulness.

64. Mindful Eating

A student does not like a lesson involving snacks? Students will strive to be more conscious of what they are consuming with this innovative awareness practice.

65. Smiling Minds App

Try this free mindfulness software for kids and your students to learn fast mediation and other activities.

66. Mindful Gratitude Exercise

As students strive to be aware of what they are thankful for, they will find more contentment in their lives.

67. Quiet Time

Adding a little quiet time to the classroom schedule will allow students opportunities to reflect and concentrate on the moment.

68. Nature Walk

Embark on an active stroll to inspire the students to experience all five of their senses.

69. What Mood Are You Generating in Others?

Using this lesson plan as a reference, explore with your students how ordinary behaviors impact your peers and what they should do to bring themselves to a certain person's shoes.

70. Rainbow Bubble Breathing Story

For younger students, this "plot" of a rainbow bubble may be a perfect image to practice guided breathing.

71. Mindfulness Scavenger Hunt

When students check each box in this updated scavenger hunt, they will be moving closer and closer to exercising mindfulness.

72. Guided Meditation

Showing your little learners how to meditate can be tough. You can help them learn how, with this guided meditation, designed for children.

73. Mindfulness Safari
In this mindfulness safari, you will benefit from the safety of your schoolyard to pay heed to the environment around you.

74. Positive Affirmations
Check out this collection of 125 optimistic mantras that your students should use when meditating or focusing on their abilities.

75. Mindful Listening
Listening is a very necessary aspect of mindfulness. Using this tool to teach the students how to become attentive listeners at school and elsewhere.

76. Build a Face Story Stones
This exercise will help students know how to identify and understand various emotions.

77. Blindfolded Taste Test
Taste is a strong feeling, and this practice may be especially useful for helping students to recognize various sensations.

78. Mindful or Unmindful? Worksheet
To make sure the students recognize what mindfulness is and isn't, fill out this workbook as a lesson.

79. Being Mindful of Anger
Anger can be difficult for children to process, and even harder to react to healthily. Use this quick script of meditation to help calm the students when they feel overwhelmed.

80. Mindful Journaling Prompts
Seek any of these journaling tips with older students regarding trust and self-esteem to help them focus on their inner and outer encounters.

81. Read a Book About Mindfulness
Learn aloud with this collection of 11 best books on literacy for young

students from Learn Brilliantly.

82. Who Am I? Game
This popular game teaches students to be vigilant and make discoveries, which can help improve knowledge.

83. Emotion Octopus Craft
Learning about our feelings has never seemed so adorable! Let each child put an emotional octopus together, and then have a class discussion about feelings.

84. Today I Feel
In your school, put up this Muppet-themed poster and show students how to understand the feelings they experience every day.

85. Square Breaths
Square relaxation is a quick and efficient approach to help relax students when they feel stressed.

86. Finding Silver Linings
Mindfulness involves just as much analysis as observation does. This activity teaches students how to reframe negative experiences and learn from them.

87. Body Scan
Try this fast body scanning meditation as a class to concentrate on emotions and sensations

88. Assessing vs. Judging Others
Do you know the difference between looking at another person and judging them? Teach your students how to use this social-emotional learning activity to assess others carefully.

89. Pause and Think Online
Mindfulness should be a big aspect of teaching healthy global citizenship! This Common Sense Media activity shows the students how to pause before reacting to something online.

90. Freeze Dance Mindfulness
Make a freeze dance party for your teacher as a pleasant way to involve the students and educate them about being conscious.

91. What Are You Doing? Activity

This practice shows all students how to listen attentively and pay more attention to their acts.

92. Stop and Think Worksheet

Any action that we take may cause a positive or negative reaction in others. Send this worksheet to your pupils, then explore why it's necessary to acknowledge the reactions of others.

93. Raisin Exercise

Offer each pupil a raisin, and then practice examining it utilizing each of the five senses. The Greater Good Science Center at Berkeley recommends doing this exercise multiple times in order to get the full effect but even once can be a useful experience for your students.

94. Red Light, Green Light

It is a great game, P.E. Staple, but did you know you can use it to teach observation — a core part of your conscience?

95. Loving Kindness Meditation

Love meditations of empathy help one to show respect for others — a beautiful combination of mindfulness and student social-emotional development.

96. Root to Rising Activity

Each program incorporates relaxation and reflection to enable students to cultivate self-assurance and harmony actively.

97. Draw Your Breath

This art activity will help students develop breadth sensitivity and use the experience to transfer to relaxation.

98. Melt or Freeze?

Mindfulness is a perfect opportunity for the students to control their urges. This exercise makes the students sort between impulsive ("melt") and conscientious ("freeze") acts.

99. Rainbow Walk

Go for a stroll with your students and inspire them to find the red, orange, yellow, green, blue, indigo, and purple as a simple way to exercise mindfulness.

100. Tuning into Different Moods
If we are tired or distracted, it can be hard to recall to be aware of our emotions. This task takes only a few minutes while you instruct students to consider what they're thinking at the moment.

101. Emotions Bottles
Although we don't encourage students to "bottle up" their thoughts, this exercise incorporates the Inside Out Pixar video to understand their emotions.

THE MINDFULNESS AND KIDS WHO LEARN AND THINK DIFFERENTLY

The effects of teaching children to be conscious have been attracting publicity. Studies have shown that it can help children improve their behavior and focus. Some schools have even begun to train thoughtfulness in the classroom.

Improved behavior and focus is a plus for all children. But it can be even more valuable to children who learn and think differently. This is especially true of children who are anxious or impulsive.

Even children failing in school can have adverse interactions that may contribute to pessimistic thought. These experiences can reduce their motivation and make them feel defeated. Being willing to recognize and remove such destructive emotions will help children remain concentrated and optimistic. This will also bring a sense of calm.

Practicing Mindfulness
Mindfulness will not automatically apply to most youngsters. However, it can be taught. There are some online learning tools and books (for children and adults), so you can help your child learn at home. You can also find coachings in your area. And there are thoughtfulness and calming applications for babies.

Practicing Mindfulness typically requires meditation techniques. The aim is to concentrate on every step, in and out. In a classroom setting, the instructor may encourage children to notice when their minds wander and gently remind them to bring their thoughts back to their breathing sensations.

Younger children can be offered a stuffed toy to put on their chest. Seeing it rise and fall allows things more clear to concentrate on breathing.

However, your child doesn't need to take classes to learn mindfulness. You can also try exercises like this at home. Have in mind that focusing on your breath can be harder than it sounds to be, especially for kids who need your attention.

There are, indeed, avenues to incorporate relaxation outside of meditation exercises. For example, children can try to see how their body feels, or how their feet connect with the floor and their seats to the chairs. You can also practice being mindful while you're moving, so kids don't have to sit down.

Here Are Other Ways You Can Work On It At Home:
• Search for children's books on what it takes to concentrate on the moment and how to learn peaceful breathing. Choose a book that suits your child's age to share.
• A model of mindfulness for your child. Point out times when you're using mindfulness to control anxiety or emotions.
• When children seem anxious, encourage them to stop doing what they're doing for a minute and notice what they're feeling.

Mindfulness does not aid kids only in the short term period. It also helps them build long-term strength.
When children discovered that their thoughts drifting and then bring their attention back to the breath, it will help them build focus. Every time they catch themselves before reacting to something they think about, it will assist them in build self-control. Mindfulness can also assist kids to become more self-aware and benefit self-esteem.

HOW CAN MINDFULNESS HELP PARENTS MAINTAIN BETTER RELATIONSHIPS WITH THEIR CHILDREN?

Youth can be a stressful period in the relationship between parent and child. Can mindfulness help? A new pilot study has taken an innovative approach to the problem, which combines both preteen and parent classes with parent brain scans and reports from their children on how mother or dad did.

Previous studies have shown that consciousness practice can reduce stress, depression, and anxiety in pre-school and disabled parents — and that conscious parental care is associated with positive children's behavior. This new study is the first to use neural imagery to see how consciousness changes parents' brains — and the results suggest that cultivating awareness every moment may make them calmer and more empathetic to their children.

The study led by Elliot T. Berkman from the University of Oregon consisted of 18 parent-and-child pairs. Each pair took a week-old Mindful Families Stress Reduction Course, which was designed by Jone Kabat-Zinn, Professor Emeritus at the University of Massachusetts Medical School, to adapt the gold standard Mindfulness-Based Stress Reduction course.

Importantly, there was no explicit parenting instruction in these sessions. "It just came together and practiced a variety of exercises," said Lisa May, the study's first author. "There is one popular in which everybody gets a raisin, and everybody sees enjoys it."

Parents and children were often sent home with several organized yoga exercises, including an activity that required to concentrate on brushing their teeth carefully. Not every family has been very diligent in doing outside the weekly courses, but this isn't necessarily a bad thing. "I consider that partly speaks of being a busy person and even more promising results," said May.

The researchers used functional magnetic resonance imaging (fMRI) before and after the course to look into the neural activity in their parents' brains while they were exercising careful breathing and when their minds were asked to walk. Parents and children also completed pre- and post-course surveys.

Overall, after completing the course, parents experience reduced tension and improved understanding. And there was a relationship between the two — parents who increased their attention most by measures showed the greatest decreases in stress. While overall adolescents have not reported a significant change in their positive view of their family relationship, overall perceptions of children that their parents pay care to them have increased significantly (so-called parental surveillance).

When May and his colleagues were contrasting the patterns of brain function in parents during the respiratory challenge and the process of roaming about their brains, the focus operation contributed to greater stimulation of brain areas that were considered to require concentration, of line with previous studies on the impact of focus on the brain.

"Instead what was more interesting was that as we looked at what moves relative to the post-intervention, we often found something entirely different: we discovered places linked to emotional health," says May. The regions that, after completion, showed increasing activity was known to involve self-awareness (precautionary and ventromedial prefrontal cortex), emotional regulation (lateral prefrontal cortex), and emotional awareness (mid-insulas). But perhaps the most interesting result in this research was that parents who had the most stimulation in a section of the brain involved in empathy and emotional regulation (the left anterior/inferior frontal gyrus) had children who considered their connection between parents and children to be more enhanced.

While tentative, these studies indicate that even attending this short course with their children has modified parents' minds and could have made them more empathetic and capable of understanding and controlling their own emotions.

"Therefore, this is really one of the great results that we often see from conscientiousness interventions, and often people say they can better display with their own emotions," says May. "For instance, these could better say, 'Oh wow, I'm upset right now,' and they simply watch these emotions rather than trying to stop themselves by eating cookies or watching it.

May stress that it is important to be careful when interpreting this small pilot study, especially since a control group is lacking. It could be the advantages of this study because parents and teenagers spend quality time together weekly.

"Parents often reported a lot of benefits derived, and their kids have reported that they also benefit from going alone with their parent once a week," Mary says. "It's wonderful in and of itself. If we were to create a tightly controlled design, we could see that fewer of these effects relate to the practice of mindfulness and more to parenting and children.

MINDFUL PARENTING KEEP KIDS OUT OF TROUBLE

Mindfulness has been a means to enhance the well-being of the person, from our wellbeing to our joy and resilience. According to critics, however, some practitioners of consciousness focus too much on self-improvement until they are absorbed. Now, two new studies are painting a different picture, suggesting that attention can help to improve others' well-being—especially our children—if we practice it.

In a study, researchers at the University of Vermont have surveyed more than 600 parents between 3 and 17 years of age to see how attention is being paid to the wellbeing of their children. Parents have reported on their attentiveness (the awareness in everyday interactions), their attention to parenting (how attentive, non-judging, and non-responsive they interact with their children), and they're positive against adverse parenting (e.g., expression of unconditional love and limitations against harsh physical penalties). They also reflected on the typical styles of coping for their children — if they tend to become anxious, depressed, or disturbed, such as hitting or shouting in difficult circumstances.

Analyzes also found that parents with more attention participate in more constructive and fewer pessimistic parenting behavior, which is related to more healthy activity, causing reduced fear, stress, and intervention.

"Conscious of your connections with your kid, and your understanding seems to prepare the way for you to become a successful father," says Justin Father, lead writer of the report.

Interestingly, parents that were merely more conscientious did not have any improved effects for their babies, indicating that being vigilant and becoming a good parent may be two separate items. Parent indicates that you can raise your sensitivity and that the discomfort, but this does not automatically mean that you should implement such skills in more stressful situations.

"It can be really difficult to alter as you establish life long habits toward your kids," he says.

Although the research by Parent shows that good, conscientious discipline is related to successful outcomes for infants, it is challenging to say why. He considers your own emotions in dispute with your child and knows to hesitate, sometimes in disagreement, before answering with frustration, and listening carefully to the perspective of a kid. Such skills may help maintain the bond between parent and infant, while also helping to model how to manage challenging circumstances.

In another recent research, Caitlin Turpin and Tara Chaplin of George Mason University have attempted to explore this relation by placing parents and children in the laboratory in order to look into their real-time contact.

Here, parents who had registered on a degree of cautious childhood were asked to address the complicated tension in their relationships with their 12- to 14-year-old daughters. This discussion has been recorded and analyzed to display how many parents share their kids with their positive emotions, negative emotions, and positive feelings as well. These results were then compared to the sexual behavior and drug use reported by the adolescent.

In their analysis, the researchers found that parents with higher conscious parenthood showed less negative emotions and more positive emotions in the conversations with their children than those who have less conscious parenthood. Bearing more optimistic feelings was, in effect, correlated with decreased children's medicine (through sexual activity was not decreased).

"Although you are a kid, loving discipline works and easy-going behavior works," Chaplin notes.

Interestingly, positive or negative expressions of emotions alone seem to make little difference in adolescent sex or drug use, although previous studies have linked the negative of a parent to adolescent risk-taking. Chaplin speculates that it is probably more critical than a parent is emotionally responsive to its infant than that in the experiences it is either optimistic or negatively.

"Cautious childhood can be more focus with harmony or emotional congruence on the interaction, not just parents who show love a lot," she says. It would not even be really helpful to show affections through stressful discussions.

Taken together, these findings suggest that promoting more compassionate, sensitive parenting – and lower discipline or yelling – can implicitly help children escape adolescence dangers, such as depression, anxiety, behavior, and drug usage. Chaplin believes that caring parenthood helps, as parents are linked to their parenting goals.

"Guardian often want to do the right thing when they are Guarding their kids. They want to be warm, structure, rules, consequences and all these are good things," said Chaplin. "But most times they stumble when their young girl slams the door angrily in her face. That is where conscientious discipline fits in.

The studies of both Chaplin and Parent are just preliminary and do not necessarily demonstrate that careful parenting causes the measured effects. There might be other theories behind their observations. For starters, proactive parenting will strengthen the partnership of the parent with his or her spouse, which another Parent research indicates and which may explain for a successful child coping. This may also be accurate if the dynamic is inverted, which implies that a parent 's desire to behave more wisely affects the issues of children.

Both researchers recognize this and say that further studies are necessary. Parent wants to delineate further how attentive parenting affects children's emotional regulation. Chaplin is conducting a randomized, regulated trial that contrasts an 8-week diligent parenting course to a traditional parenting course and tests how this impacts the relationships between parents and children. They hope that their work can finally show that loving parentage is a valuable tool to support parents and their babies.

"I have zero knowledge we still know sufficient about it. But if we demonstrate that our programs increase parental awareness and reduce the risk behavior of their teens, we would be more sure that it is a parental responsibility, "says Chaplin. "And both Guardian will have to carry it out."

INSTRUCTIONS AND RECOMMENDATIONS

Listen With Your Child

For kids (especially children under the age of ten), it's important to listen to new instructions meditation with mature minds, at least the first few times. I always suggest a few basic questions during each mediation session: How did you feel while we were doing the mediation? Which part did you like best? Didn't you like anything about it? Start posing questions like these to get a feel of how the child is reacting to the exercise through time.

If the meditations resonate with your child or students, after they have become comfortable with you, they can use them on their own. Kids may also choose to practice meditation after a while without the recordings. If they continue to practice alone — with or without the guided meditations — I recommend that you keep checking in with them, asking questions about how it goes.

Use Speakers, Not Headphones

We help children learn to be involved in their world, and headphones may lead them to feel cut off from their surroundings, so listening via a speaker is preferred. There are exceptions for this especially: it happens in situations where there are a lot of distractions and you will need to be the judge of whether headphones are a better choice.

Meditating With Eyes Open Is Okay!

Children should never be pressured to close their eyes unless they are at ease to do so. Many people have a preconceived notion that when we meditate, our eyes should be closed, but in all my meditations documented, I offer the choice of open or closed eyes. Neither is automatically more successful, and this is valid for both children and adults (in my own practice, I meditate around half the time with my eyes open). With eyes closed and open, our perspectives may be different, and it's nice if the children feel confident doing both.

Meditation Should Not Be Mandatory

For two important reasons, meditation practice can't be treated like homework or music practice. First, it's an entirely internal experience, so if children are to succeed, they need to be self-motivated and interested. Second, requiring a child to practice meditation is essentially useless, because you can not control the inner life of someone else — nor can you have direct proof of that. Without meditating at all, children can sit quietly for five minutes, and you won't necessarily know what kind of experience they have. The best you can do is offer circumstances in which an experienced child can discover the benefits. The interest of children must lead them and guide the amount of time they spend doing meditation. They may want to practice one day, not the next, or they may lose interest on one occasion for weeks or months. As difficult as this may be for parents, it is my strong recommendation that you offer your support and gently suggest that they try meditation but never require them to do so, especially when you encounter resistance.

Mindfulness Is Not About Calming Down

While meditation sometimes calms us down (and we always want kids to calm down!), it's crucial to note that the aim of meditation on mindfulness is simply to be conscious of how one feels at this moment. We want to provide children with the "room" to feel nervous, anxious, or excited — and to become aware of their feelings. Paradoxically, negative emotions are generally understood and embraced, resulting in greater peace. Yet that's not the purpose of wanting to cool down, so it may potentially trigger fear and be detrimental. The intention should be to accept the moment as it is, even uncomfortable feelings. For example, when kids feel restless, we hope they can answer by thinking something like: It's really hard to sit still right now, and that's OK. Often, everyone thinks this way. I can get curious about how I feel, take a breath, notice my body's energy and sensations, listen to sounds, and be OK.

Your Practice Comes First

In the long term, I think modeling is the most important thing you can do to maintain a child's interest in meditation. I recommend you let your children witness your regular practice, or at least be aware of it. Talk about how meditation benefits you from time to time, or what you find interesting about it — especially when it's relevant to something that comes up in your life. You can even consider meditating in a space where your kids are engaging in some tasks for a few minutes. Set a timer and let them know you'll sit down and meditate for five minutes while they're playing or reading. They might surprise you every once in a while by asking questions about what you're doing — or even sit down and join in! But whether they practice it or not, watching the adults practicing meditation in their lives has a significant effect on the babies.

YOGA FOR KIDS: TORMENT OF A SILENT MIND

Why is Yoga even more popular with children today than it was yesterday? Well, kids are just as likely to be stressed as adults are. How could a lot of this be asking? Kids' pressure comes from additional education requirements (like more homework) We all know how important it is to further our child's education to give them a better chance of life, but when life can be destroyed, it's time to take action.

Yoga for children is a beautiful blessing to send to a kid who wants peace of mind. Pressure placed on our children today can be exacerbated by certain causes, such as being harassed. Children also suffer at the hands of their parents while watching them worry about debt or anything that comes with surviving in the 21st century. How can we help the mind of a tormented child, simply introduce it to Yoga?

Children's yoga allows children to become conscious of the body and to begin to realize how important it is to keep children in good health. Even at an early age, children need to develop better body awareness, and after doing so, they take control of themselves to lead an active, healthy life. Children who perform yoga self-educate themselves to self-control strength and synchronization.

Exercises for adolescents have been found to help calm down Overly aggressive activities in certain situations. Yoga helped children by positively channeling their impulses. Yoga moves for minors are just as different from the way adults practice. A couple of poses for children that work perfectly well are the Warrior Pose and the Tree Pose. Both are exercises that help the child find calm, build trust and balance.

Some children go back to yoga like ducks' mud, whilst others have to be coaxed and require encouragement and the advantages pointing out. The trick to having a suspicious child to participate in a yoga class is to illustrate how it's a common craze among other children. Point out how much fun this can be. Explain the details of the Warrior posture that moves in your quest to encourage the child. Ease their pain if you're scared to do yoga on your own. Let them know that they can team up with a partner, which will also help build on their team skills and thus gain a bond with others.

There will be times when children find it difficult to focus and concentrate, but this is not the case with all children, whether they practice yoga or not. Kids and rest are not compatible. Just having a child close his eyes for a while will be a task in his self. Ask the child to visualize something he/she is interested in or enjoy doing.

Try them with your belly, breathing yoga exercise while listening to relaxing music. Ask them to imagine they 're floating up in space or making sandcastles on the beach. After the session is over, invite the child to share their experience of how they felt while practicing the Kids Yoga routine.

If they reveal their secret thoughts, this can only mean that the child has opened up, and what a major breakthrough it is. It's enough to have your child share a secret to say they want to be heard.

The quiet feelings that once plagued your little boy/girl will give you, as a loving adult, insight into how to cope with what was once a tormented, empty mind.

Children's yoga is the wealthiest form of knowledge for any child.

MYTHS AND FACTS ABOUT MINDFULNESS FOR KIDS

Myth 1: Mindfulness Is Just Sitting Silently.

Meditation is one form of exercising morality, although several other elements and methods of doing so are available. Explore all sorts of practices to find the ones that best work for you! There are two examples.

• **Positive Movement:** Seek meditation, tai chi, or simply to stroll with awareness.

• **Patient eating/dinner:** Pick a snack or meal and consume very gradually, taking note of the appearance and flavor.

Myth 2: Mindfulness Is Religious.
Skills in mindfulness are focused on the ability to concentrate on the air. We all smoke all the time, so breathing influences the body physiologically. Slow deep breathing may reduce heart rate and blood pressure, whereas fast quick breathing can have a reverse effect. Treatment is focused on neuroscience. If in the school setting, parental education may be appropriate.

Myth 3: "I Don't Have Time For Mindfulness."
It is a global recommendation that in order to coach mindfulness, you should also be engaged in mindfulness yourself. Integrate it into your day to day activities by taking just a few minutes each day to meditate and focus to your breath. Also, consider one activity you do daily that you could do more mindfully, perhaps, driving or brushing your teeth. You may choose to use an app to help you get started; for this set aside Five-Ten minutes every day.

Note: if you are brand new to practicing mindfulness, it may be harder than it sounds! When I first started carrying out the activities, I was amazed at how frequently throughout my day, I was not mindful. There was a realization that this was an area of development I did not even know it was needed.
Just have in mind that part of mindful is kind and non-judgmental, accept yourself wherever you are, and know that it is worth the effort.

How To Achieve Mindfulness Into The School Daily Activities With Students
Start by integrating one-minute intervals of meditations throughout the day. You may also need to add mindfulness-based journal prompts to your daily activities, read a kids' book about mindfulness, or add a kindness jar to your class. Research has shown that mindfulness in the classroom can result in increased teaching time (Mindful Life Project, 2016) and improved teaching efficacy (Meiklejohn et al. 2012).

Myth 4: "I Do Not Have The Financial Resources Mindfulness To Implement Into My Classroom."
Breathing free! If it is not financial, breathwork can still be integrated into the regular school day. There are free online resources, such as Every Moment Counts: Quiet Moments Card Program. This program is a built-in program to promote the positive mental health of students by providing a way to respond to situational stress throughout the day.
If you are a teacher or administrator seeking a full curriculum range, you may want to consider Mind Up, The Hawn Foundation.

Myth 5: There Is A Lack Of Evidence To Mindfulness With Children.
While it is true that high-quality research is needed to awareness with children, the research that is out there is very promising, and a recent meta-analysis (Dunning et al., 2019) does not support the use of consciousness-based interventions to improve mental health and well-being of children. Also, there is no risk related to practice mindfulness. mindfulness practices to teach coping strategies to help with self-regulation.

Myth 6: Children Do Not Need Attention.
The term "positive mental health" recognized that health is more than the absence of disease, and we all have mental health as we all have physical health. Having positive mental health means that one can engage in productive activities and have the ability to utilize coping skills.

According to the mental health of children is the latest (Child Mind Institute, 2018):

- 30% of kids are affected by anxiety at one point or another.
- There has been a 17% increase in anxiety over the past ten years.
- 80% of those affected by anxiety never receive proper treatment. Only 1% seek treatment in the year symptoms begins.
- Untreated anxiety disorders are associated with an increased risk for depression, school failure, and substance abuse.

All kids need mental health promotion, and mindfulness is a tool to do so.

Myth 7: Kids Would Not Like Mindfulness.
Mindfulness activities for children should be fun! In my experience, they do enjoy it. Each of us may have mindfulness practices we like, and ones do not like it. So, do not be discouraged if students do not like to exercise or activity your first try.

Mindfulness can be implemented with children in many ways. Take the time to have them only see their breath, and then take a couple of deep breaths. Make more fun with spinning pinwheels with your breath or make crafts dragon breathing "fire" through.

Myth 8: Mindfulness Lacks Evidence And Research And Therefore Shouldn't Be Used In The Classroom.

Fact: There is an extensive amount of research on the utility of mindfulness practices for decreasing symptoms of stress, anxiety, depression, and improving pro-social behavior such as empathy, perspective-taking, and attention.

Myth: Mindfulness and other social-emotional learning activities trends take time away from the curriculum.
Fact: Mindfulness strategies can easily be built into the curriculum. Remember, it only involves a moment to moment awareness of what you experience without judgment. These aspects can be built into the curriculum naturally, and thus potentially improving the student experience.

Myth 9: Teacher Can not Use Mindfulness If They Do not Attend Training
Fact: You can combine multiple techniques into your class consciousness without attending expensive training. However, commensurate with any exercise, you should be sure to practice only within your limits. Thus, teachers should not be practicing deep meditation, or process the trauma or mental health problem using the procedures of awareness in the classroom. Instead, simple guided breathing exercises can be accessed by all levels of practitioners.

Myth: Mindfulness is only for children who have experienced trauma or have significant behavioral problems.
Fact: Everyone can benefit from a little attention! It offers a way for you to be present with your experience, and some of the principles of good manners on how to approach life and interactions with others. For individuals with trauma, and depending on the importance of behavioral problems exhibited, it may be more appropriate to refer or consult a mental health professional.

Myth 10: It Takes Time For Busy Teachers To Learn Mindfulness.
Fact: Well, it's a good excuse to practice mindfulness! Mindfulness has been shown to decrease the negative effects of stress. Exercising attention will not only allow you to use it with students; it likely will positively impact your ability to cope with the large stress of being a teacher. Of course, many people choose to deepen their practice in awareness by studying extensively, taking courses, attending conferences, etc. However, people just need to do as much appropriate for themselves and their goals today.

While interesting, teaching, and learning in the school community can also be stressful. Interest using a growing awareness in educational settings, such as the body of research to support its use for reducing toxic stress and increase pro-social behavior. Hopefully, you can pick up a few pieces of awareness in your daily instructional practices to help you and your students enjoy the school year and reduce your reactivity to stress that detracts from the learning process.

CONCLUSION

Children of all ages can benefit from awareness, the simple practice brings a gentle attitude, accept for the moment. It can help parents and caregivers as well, to promote happiness and eliminate stress. Here, we offer basic tips for children and adults of all ages, as well as some of the activities that develop compassion, focus, curiosity, and empathy. And remember, the attention can be fun.

The difficulty comes to us from the moment we were born. Babies get hungry and tired. Toddlers wrestle with the language and self-control. And as children develop through adolescence into adolescence, life grows increasingly complicated. Develop relationships, navigation school, and exercise independence - very terms of growth - naturally create a stressful situation for each child.

At each stage of development, awareness can be a useful tool to reduce anxiety and promote happiness. Mindfulness - a simple technique that emphasizes the attention to this point in accepting, non-judgmental way - has emerged as a major practice popular in recent decades. It is taught to executives in companies, athletes in the locker room, and more, for children both at home and at school.

Children are uniquely suited to benefit from the practice of mindfulness. Habits formed in early life will inform behavior in adulthood, and with awareness, we have the opportunity to give our children the habit of peaceful, good, and receive.

"For children, attention can offer relief from whatever difficulties they may face in life," said Annaka Harris, an author who teaches awareness to children. "It also gives them the beauty of being in the moment."

Part of the reason why attention is very effective for children can be explained by the way the brain develops. While our brains continue to develop throughout our lives, connections in the prefrontal circuits are created at their fastest rate during childhood. Mindfulness, which promotes skills that are controlled in the prefrontal cortex, such as focus and cognitive control, could, therefore, have a special impact on the development of skills, including self-regulation, judgment, and patience during childhood.

Do Not Go Yet; One Last Thing To Do
 If you enjoyed this book or found it useful, I'd be very grateful if you'd post a short review on Amazon. Your support does make a difference, and I read all the reviews personally so I can get your feedback and make this book even better.
Thanks for your help and support!